LOW GLYCEMIC INDEX

COOKBOOK

FOR

NEWBIES AND BEGINNERS

BY

Dr. Christen Zimmermann

Table of Contents

INTRODUCTION

A glycemic index diet is an eating plan based on how foods affect your blood sugar level. The glycemic index is a system of assigning a number to carbohydrate-containing foods according to how much each food increases blood sugar. The glycemic index itself is not a diet plan but one of various tools — such as calorie counting or carbohydrate counting — for guiding food choices.

The term "glycemic index diet" usually refers to a specific diet plan that uses the index as the primary or only guide for meal planning. Unlike some other plans, a glycemic index diet doesn't necessarily specify portion sizes or the optimal number of calories, carbohydrates, or fats for weight loss or weight maintenance. Many popular commercial diets, diet books and diet websites are based on the glycemic index, including the Zone Diet, Sugar Busters and the Slow-Carb Diet.

Purpose

The purpose of a glycemic index (GI) diet is to eat carbohydrate-containing foods that are less likely to cause large increases in blood sugar levels. The diet could be a means to lose weight and prevent chronic diseases related to obesity such as diabetes and cardiovascular disease.

Why you might follow the GI diet

You might choose to follow the GI diet because you:

• Want to lose weight or maintain a healthy weight

• Need help planning and eating healthier meals

• Need help maintaining blood sugar levels as part of a diabetes treatment plan

Studies suggest that a GI diet can help achieve these goals. However, you might be able to achieve the same health benefits by eating a healthy diet, maintaining a healthy weight and getting enough exercise. Check with your doctor or health care provider before starting any weight-loss diet, especially if you have any health conditions, including diabetes.

THE GLYCEMIC INDEX

The GI principle was first developed as a strategy for guiding food choices for people with diabetes. An international GI database is maintained by Sydney

University Glycemic Index Research Services in Sydney, Australia. The database contains the results of studies conducted there and at other research facilities around the world. A basic overview of carbohydrates, blood sugar and GI values is helpful for understanding glycemic index diets.

Carbohydrates

Carbohydrates, or carbs, are a type of nutrient in foods. The three basic forms are sugars, starches and fiber. When you eat or drink something with carbs, your body breaks down the sugars and starches into a type of sugar called glucose, the main source of energy for cells in your body. Fiber passes through your body undigested. Two main hormones from your pancreas help regulate glucose in your bloodstream. The hormone insulin moves glucose from your blood into your cells. The hormone glucagon helps release glucose stored in your liver when your blood sugar (blood glucose) level is low. This process helps keep your body fueled and ensures a natural balance in blood glucose.

Different types of carbohydrate foods have properties that affect how quickly your body digests them and how quickly glucose enters your bloodstream.

UNDERSTANDING GI VALUES

There are various research methods for assigning a GI value to food. In general, the number is based on how much a food item raises blood glucose levels compared with how much pure glucose raises blood glucose. GI values are generally divided into three categories:

• Low GI: 1 to 55

• Medium GI: 56 to 6

• High GI: 70 and higher

Comparing these values, therefore, can help guide healthier food choices. For example, an English muffin made with white wheat flour has a GI value of 77. A whole-wheat English muffin has a GI value of 45.

LIMITATIONS OF GI VALUES

One limitation of GI values is that they don't reflect the likely quantity you would eat of a particular food. For example, watermelon has a GI value of 80, which would put it in the category of food to avoid. But watermelon has relatively few digestible carbohydrates in a typical serving. In other words, you have to eat a lot of watermelon to significantly raise your blood glucose level.

To address this problem, researchers have developed the idea of glycemic load (GL), a numerical value hat indicates the change in blood glucose levels when you eat a typical serving of the food. For example, a 4.2-ounce (120-gram, or 3/4-cup) serving of watermelon has a GL value of 5, which would identify it as a healthy food choice. For comparison, a 2.8-ounce (80-gram, or 2/3-cup) serving of raw carrots has a GL value of 2.

Other issues

A GI value tells us nothing about other nutritional information. For example, whole milk has a GI value of 31 and a GL value of 4 for a 1-cup (250-milliliter) serving. But because of its high fat content, whole milk is not the best choice for weight loss or weight control.

The published GI database is not an exhaustive list of foods, but a list of those foods that have been studied.

Many healthy foods with low GI values are not in the database.

The GI value of any food item is affected by several factors, including how the food is prepared, how it is processed and what other foods are eaten at the same time.

Also, there can be a range in GI values for the same foods, and some would argue it makes it an unreliable guide to determine food choices.

CRAB-STUFFED AVOCADOS

Stuffing the cavity of a halved avocado has to be one of the easiest ways to serve it, and this crab filling can be made ahead

Ingredients

• 100g white crabmeat

• 1 tsp Dijon mustard

• 2 tbsp olive oil

• handful basil leaves, shredded with a few of the smaller leaves left whole, to serve

• 1 red chilli , deseeded and chopped

• 2 avocados

Method

• STEP 1

To make the crab mix, flake the crabmeat into a small bowl and mix in the mustard and oil, then season to taste.

Can be made the day ahead. Add the basil and chilli just before serving.

• STEP 2

To serve, halve and stone the avocados. Fill each cavity with a quarter of the crab mix, scatter with a few of the smaller basil leaves and eat with teaspoons.

CHICKEN WITH CRUSHED HARISSA CHICKPEAS

Need something speedy for dinner? Try this chicken, coated in flavourful za'atar and served with spiced chickpeas. It's simple, but seriously delicious

Ingredients

- 2 tbsp rapeseed oil

- 1 onion , chopped

- 1 red pepper , finely sliced

- 1 yellow pepper , finely sliced

- 4 chicken breasts

- 1 tbsp za'atar

- 400g can chickpeas

- 1½ tbsp red harissa paste

- 150g baby spinach

- ½ small bunch of parsley , finely chopped

- lemon wedges, to serve

Method

• Heat 1 tbsp of oil in a frying pan over a medium heat and fry the onions and peppers for 7 mins until softened and golden.

• Meanwhile, put the chicken between two sheets of baking parchment and lightly bash until about 2cm thick. Mix together the remaining oil and the za'atar, then rub over the chicken. Season to taste.

• Heat the grill to high. Put the chicken on a baking tray lined with foil, and grill for 3-4 mins each side, or until golden and cooked through.

• Heat the chickpeas in a pan with the harissa paste and 2 tbsp water until warmed through, then roughly mash with a potato masher. Wilt the spinach in a pan with 1 tbsp of water or in the microwave in a heatproof bowl. Stir the pepper and onion mixture, spinach and parsley through the chickpeas. Serve with the sliced chicken and the lemon wedges for squeezing over.

SMOKED SALMON WITH PRAWNS, HORSERADISH CREAM & LIME VINAIGRETTE

This stunning starter can be assembled ahead, then topped with dressed leaves just before serving.

Ingredients

- 1 tbsp crème fraîche

- 1 tsp horseradish sauce

- 4 slices smoked salmon

- 10 large cooked prawns, peeled but tails left on

For the salad

- juice 1 lime, finely grated zest of ½

- 1 tsp clear honey

- ½ tsp finely grated fresh root ginger

- 2 tbsp light olive oil

- 2 handfuls small leaf salad

Method

- STEP 1

Mix the crème fraîche with the horseradish and a little salt and pepper. For the dressing, whisk the lime juice and zest with the honey, ginger and seasoning, then whisk in the oil. Lay the smoked salmon and prawns on 2 plates, then top with a dollop of the horseradish cream. Toss the salad in most of the dressing and pile on top. Drizzle the remaining dressing around the plate and serve.

CHEESY AUTUMN MUSHROOMS

A low-carb treat, ready in 5 mins

Ingredients

• 4 large field mushrooms

• 100g gorgonzola or other blue cheese , crumbled

• 25g walnuts , toasted and roughly chopped

• 4 thyme sprigs

• knob butter , cut into small pieces

• rocket leaves, to serve

Method

• STEP 1

Heat oven to 200C/fan 180C/gas 6. Arrange the mushrooms on a baking tray. Scatter over the cheese, walnuts, thyme sprigs and butter. You can do up to this stage a day in advance.

• STEP 2

Pop in the oven and cook for 10 mins until the cheese is melted and the mushrooms are softened. Arrange some rocket leaves on plates and place the mushrooms on top.

STUFFED COURGETTE ROLLS

Try Gordon Ramsay's take on Italian antipasti - tantalise your palate with this no-cook starter

Ingredients

• 4small courgettes , ends trimmed

• 3-4 tbsp olive oil , plus extra to drizzle

• 3-4 tbsp balsamic vinegar , to drizzle

• 250g tub ricotta

• squeeze lemon juice

• handful fresh basil leaves , chopped

• 50g pine nut , toasted (see Know-how, below)

Method

• STEP 1

Slice the courgettes lengthways, using a swivel vegetable peeler – you'll need 24 long strips. Drizzle some of the olive oil and balsamic over two large plates and lay the strips flat, trying not to overlap. Sprinkle with more oil and balsamic, cover and leave to marinate in the fridge for at least 20 mins. Can be prepared up to 6 hrs ahead.

• STEP 2

Mix the ricotta with lemon juice and seasoning to taste, then mix in the basil and pine nuts. Place 1 tsp of the ricotta mixture onto one end of a courgette strip and roll up. Repeat until you have used up all the filling. Arrange rolls upright on a plate and grind over some black pepper. Drizzle with a little more oil and balsamic vinegar to serve.

HEALTHY BEEF STEW

Try our easy, healthy beef stew recipe that's packed full of vitamin C. This warming dinner is perfect for chilly nights

Ingredients

• 1 onion, sliced

• 1 garlic clove, sliced

• 2 tbsp olive oil

• 300g pack beef stir-fry strips, or use beef steak, thinly sliced

• 1 yellow pepper, deseeded and thinly sliced

• 400g can chopped tomato

• sprig rosemary, chopped

• handful pitted olives

Method

• STEP 1

In a large saucepan, cook onion and garlic in olive oil for 5 mins until softened and turning golden. Tip in the beef strips, pepper, tomatoes and rosemary, then bring to the boil. Simmer for 15 mins until the meat is cooked through, adding some boiling water if needed. Stir through the olives and serve with mash or polenta.

ROASTED RATATOUILLE CHICKEN

A classic chicken recipe that will keep the crowds coming back for more

Ingredients

• 1 onion , cut into wedges

• 2 red pepper , seeded and cut into chunks

• 1 courgette , cut into chunks

• 1 small aubergine , cut into chunks

• 4 tomatoes , halved

• 4 tbsp olive oil , plus extra for drizzling

• 4 chicken breasts , skin on

• few rosemary sprigs (optional)

Method

• STEP 1

Heat oven to 200C/fan 180C/gas 6. Lay all the vegetables and the tomatoes in a shallow roasting tin. Pour over the olive oil and give everything a good mix round until well coated (hands are easiest for this).

• STEP 2

Put the chicken breasts, skin side up, on top of the vegetables and tuck in some rosemary sprigs, if using. Season everything with salt and black pepper and drizzle a little oil over the chicken. Roast for about 35 mins until the vegetables are soft and the chicken is golden. Drizzle with oil before serving.

NUTTY CHICKEN CURRY

Fast and flavoursome, this creamy chicken curry is ready in under 20 minutes

Ingredients

• 1 large red chilli , deseeded

• ½ a finger-length piece fresh root ginger , roughly chopped

• 1 fat garlic clove

• small bunch coriander , stalks roughly chopped

• 1 tbsp sunflower oil

• 4 skinless chicken breasts , cut into chunks

• 5 tbsp peanut butter

• 150ml chicken stock

• 200g tub Greek yogurt

Method

• STEP 1

Finely slice a ⃞uarter of the chilli, then put the rest in a food processor with the ginger, garlic, coriander stalks and one-third of the leaves. Whizz to a rough paste with a splash of water if needed.

• STEP 2

Heat the oil in a frying pan, then quickly brown the chicken chunks for 1 min. Stir in the paste for another min, then add the peanut butter, stock and yogurt. When the sauce is gently bubbling, cook for 10 mins until the chicken is just cooked through and sauce thickened. Stir in most of the remaining coriander, then scatter the rest on top with the chilli, if using. Eat with rice or mashed sweet potato.

EASY CHICKEN CASSEROLE

This flavoursome, low-fat chicken casserole is easy to make and freezes really well, so why not make double and freeze for speedy midweek meals

Ingredients

• 2 tbsp sunflower oil

• 400g boneless, skinless chicken thigh , trimmed and cut into chunks

• 1 onion , finely chopped

• 3 carrots , finely chopped

• 3 celery sticks, finely chopped

• 2 thyme sprigs or ½ tsp dried

• 1 bay leaf , fresh or dried

• 600ml vegetable or chicken stock

• 2 x 400g / 14oz cans haricot beans , drained

• chopped parsley , to serve

Method

• STEP 1

Heat the oil in a large pan, add the chicken, then fry until lightly browned. Add the veg, then fry for a few mins more. Stir in the herbs and stock. Bring to the boil. Stir well, reduce the heat, then cover and cook for 40 mins, until the chicken is tender.

• STEP 2

Stir the beans into the pan, then simmer for 5 mins. Stir in the parsley and serve with crusty bread.

TUNA STEAKS WITH CUCUMBER RELISH

Good source of heart-healthy omega-3 fatty acids

Ingredients

• 3 tbsp olive oil

• 4 tuna steaks, about 140g/5oz each

For the relish

• ½ cucumber

• 2 spring onions, finely chopped

• 1 medium tomato, finely chopped

• ½ large red chilli, seeded and finely chopped

• 1tbsp olive oil

• 2tbsp chopped parsley

• 1tbsp lime or lemon juice

Method

• STEP 1

Put the oil into a food bag and add the tuna steaks. Rub well together and leave for 30 mins while you make the relish. Peel the cucumber, halve lengthways and scoop out the seeds. Chop the flesh into a small dice. Mix with the rest of the ingredients, seasoning to taste. Set aside.

• STEP 2

To griddle: heat the pan to hot, then cook the steaks, turning after 2 mins, and cooking for another 2 mins each side depending on the thickness of the steaks. Meaty fish is best served slightly 'pink'. Remove the steaks from the heat allow to stand for 3-5 mins, then spoon over the relish and serve.

STEAMED BASS WITH GARLIC & CHILLI

Try this flavour-packed, low-fat fish dish, perfect as a mid-week meal. It's full of omega 3 and counts as 1 of your 5-a-day.

Ingredients

• 2 sea bass , or other white fish fillets

• 1 green or red chilli , deseeded and finely chopped

• 1 tsp fresh root ginger

• 300g green cabbage , finely shredded

• 2 tsp sunflower oil

• 1 tsp sesame oil

• 2 garlic cloves , thinly sliced

• 2 tsp low salt soy sauce

Method

• STEP 1

Sprinkle the fish with the chilli, ginger and a little salt. Steam the cabbage for 5 mins. Lay fish on top of the cabbage and steam for a further 5 mins until cooked through.

• STEP 2

Meanwhile, heat the oils in a small pan, add the garlic and quickly cook, stirring until lightly browned. Transfer the cabbage and fish to serving plates, sprinkle each with 1 tsp of soy sauce, then pour over the garlicky oil.

BASIL & LEMON CHICKPEAS WITH MACKEREL

Good Food favourite Lesley Waters proves that healthy can be hearty - and tasty too!

Ingredients

• 3 tbsp olive oil , plus extra for drizzling

• 1 bunch spring onion , sliced

• 1 large garlic clove , crushed

• zest 1 lemon and squeeze of juice

• 2 x 400g can chickpeas , drained and rinsed

• 150ml vegetable stock

• 85g SunBlush tomato , halved

• 4 mackerel fillets, skin on

• 1 large bunch basil

Method

• STEP 1

Heat 2 tbsp oil in a large, shallow pan. Add the spring onions, garlic and lemon zest, then cook for 2 mins until the onions are tender but still very green. Add the chickpeas, then stir until well coated in the onion mixture. Lightly crush with a potato masher, then add the stock and tomatoes. Simmer for 3-4 mins or until the liquid is absorbed, then set aside to cool slightly.

• STEP 2

Meanwhile, heat the remaining oil in a large, non-stick frying pan over a medium heat. Season the mackerel fillets on both sides and fry for 3 mins each side, starting on the skin side. You'll probably need to cook these in two batches.

• STEP 3

Add the basil and a squeeze of lemon juice to the chickpeas, then season to taste. To serve, spoon the warm chickpeas onto serving plates, drizzle with a little extra olive oil and top with the mackerel fillets.

ONE-PAN SUMMER EGGS

Satisfy your hunger with this fresh and easy vegetarian supper, or brunch if you prefer

Ingredients

• 1 tbsp olive oil

• 400g courgettes (about 2 large ones), chopped into small chunks

• 200g/7oz pack cherry tomatoes , halved

• 1 garlic clove , crushed

• 2 eggs

• few basil leaves , to serve

Method

• STEP 1

Heat the oil in a non-stick frying pan, then add the courgettes. Fry for 5 mins, stirring every so often until they start to soften, add the tomatoes and garlic, then cook for a few mins more. Stir in a little seasoning, then make two gaps in the mix and crack in the eggs. Cover the pan with a lid or a sheet of foil, then cook for 2-3 mins until the eggs are done to your liking. Scatter over a few basil leaves and serve with crusty bread.

CRANBERRY PECAN BAKED APPLES

Stuffed baked apples that taste as good as they look - and they're super healthy

Ingredients

• cooking apples

• dried cranberries

• pecans , chopped or whole

• oranges , finely grated zest and juice

Method

• STEP 1

Heat oven to 200C/180C fan/gas 6. Core cooking apples, fill their centres with dried cranberries, chopped or whole pecans and the finely grated zest and juice of oranges, then bake until tender (which should take about 20 mins).

CRANACHAN

Sweet summer raspberries folded into cream flavoured with honey, whisky and toasted oatmeal - what could be more delicious?

Ingredients

- 2 tbsp medium oatmeal

- 300g fresh British raspberries

- a little caster sugar

- 350ml double cream (we used Jersey double cream)

- 2 tbsp heather honey

- 2-3 tbsp whisky, to taste

Method

- STEP 1

To toast the oatmeal, spread it out on a baking sheet and grill until it smells rich and nutty. It will not darken quickly, so use your sense of smell to tell you when it is nutty enough. Cool the oatmeal.

- STEP 2

Make a raspberry purée by crushing half the fruit and sieving. Sweeten this to taste with a little caster sugar. Whisk the double cream until just set, and stir in the honey and whisky, trying not to over-whip the cream. Taste the mix and add more of either if you feel the need.

• STEP 3

Stir in the oatmeal and whisk lightly until the mixture is just firm. Alternate layers of the cream with the remaining whole raspberries and purée in 4 serving dishes. Allow to chill slightly before eating.

SPICED APPLE PIE

Never heard 'it's as Nepalese as apple pie'? Try this classic with a twist and you'll be converted

Ingredients

• 1 ½kg apple (Braeburns or Granny Smiths are ideal)

• s🮰ueeze lemon juice

• 2 cardamom pods or pinch of ground

• 2 tbsp flour, plus extra for rolling

• 25g golden caster sugar, plus extra for sprinkling

• 500g pack shortcrust pastry

• 2 tbsp milk

Method

• STEP 1

Heat oven to 220C/fan 200C/gas 7. Peel, core and 🮰uarter the apples, then cut into 1cm slices. Toss together with the lemon juice, then dab dry with kitchen paper so that the pie isn't too watery. If you are using whole cardamom pods, split open the shell, remove the seed from inside and grind using a pestle and mortar. Mix into the apples with the flour and sugar, then toss to get everything coated.

• STEP 2

Cut away a third of the pastry to divide into two pieces. Dust a little flour over a work surface, then roll out the larger piece to roughly 28cm wide and as thick as a £1 coin. Lift the pastry up (try loosely wrapping around a rolling pin) and spread over the bottom of a 22cm pie dish. Roll out the smaller piece of pastry a little larger than the top of the pie.

• STEP 3

Pile up the apples inside and paint around the rim of the pie with milk. Lift the smaller circle of pastry on top. Press down to seal the pie, then trim around the edge of the pie with a sharp knife and discard the excess pastry. Use your fingers to indent around the pie and form a crimped edge.

• STEP 4

Make a few slits in the pastry so that steam can escape, then brush all over with milk and sprinkle with extra sugar. Bake for 20 mins, then reduce oven to 190C/fan 170C/gas 5 and cook for 50 mins-1hr until the pastry is golden and crisp. If it starts to darken too much, cover with tin foil, but make sure you cook it uncovered for the final 10 mins so that the pastry can crisp. Serve warm or cold with whipped cream, ice cream or custard.

CRANBERRY SUNRISE

The ultimate treat for all the family

Ingredients

- 10 gelatine leaves

- 200ml hot water from the kettle

- 700ml warm, smooth-style orange juice

- 700ml warm cranberry juice

Method

- STEP 1

Soak the gelatine leaves in cold water. Drain, squeeze and dissolve the soaked gelatine in the hot water from the kettle. Add to the warm, smooth-style orange juice and set aside. Repeat the process using warm cranberry juice. Pour half of the orange juice into a large jelly mould and chill in the fridge until set completely – about 4 hours. Cover the orange jelly with half the cranberry juice and chill to set. Repeat the process until both juices are used. Leave to set overnight.

APRICOT & RASPBERRY TART

Delicious served hot or cold, this tart uses filo pastry to keep the calories down

Ingredients

- 3 large sheets filo pastry (or 6 small)

- 2 tbsp butter , melted

- 3 tbsp apricot conserve

- 6 ripe apricots , stoned and roughly sliced

- 85g raspberries

- 2 tsp caster sugar

Method

- STEP 1

Let the filo come to room temperature for about 10 mins before use. Put a baking tray into the oven and heat oven to 200C/180C fan/gas 6.

- STEP 2

Brush each large sheet of filo with melted butter, layer on top of each other, then fold in half so you have a smaller rectangle 6 layers thick. If using small sheets just stack on top of each other. Fold in the edges of the pastry base to make a 2cm border, then spread the apricot conserve inside the border. Carefully slide the pastry base on to the hot baking tray and bake for 5 mins.

• STEP 3

Remove from oven, arrange apricots over the tart and brush with any leftover melted butter. Bake for another 10 mins, then scatter on raspberries and sprinkle with sugar. Bake for a final 10 mins until the pastry is golden brown and crisp.

SPICY MEATBALLS WITH CHILLI BLACK BEANS

Give your favourite meatballs a healthy makeover with this low fat, low calorie, low GI recipe with turkey mince, black beans and avocado

Ingredients

• 1 red onion, halved and sliced

• 2 garlic cloves, sliced

• 1 large yellow pepper, quartered, deseeded and diced

• 1 tsp ground cumin

• 2-3 tsp chipotle chilli paste

• 300ml reduced-salt chicken stock

• 400g can cherry tomatoes

• 400g can black beans or red kidney beans, drained

• 1 avocado, stoned, peeled and chopped

• juice ½ lime

For the meatballs

- 500g pack turkey breast mince

- 50g porridge oats

- 2 spring onions, finely chopped

- 1 tsp ground cumin

- 1 tsp coriander

- small bunch coriander, chopped, stalks and leaves kept separate

- 1 tsp rapeseed oil

Method

- STEP 1

First make the meatballs. Tip the mince into a bowl, add the oats, spring onions, spices and the coriander stalks, then lightly knead the ingredients together until well mixed. Shape into 12 ping-pong- sized balls. Heat the oil in a non-stick frying pan, add the meatballs and cook, turning them frequently, until golden. Remove from the pan.

- STEP 2

Tip the onion and garlic into the pan with the pepper and stir-fry until softened. Stir in the cumin and chilli paste, then pour in the stock. Return the meatballs to the pan and cook, covered, over a low heat for 10 mins. Stir in the tomatoes and beans, and cook, uncovered, for a few mins more. Toss the avocado chunks in the lime juice and serve the meatballs topped with the avocado and coriander leaves.

OLD DELHI-STYLE BUTTER CHICKEN

Head to your spice rack to make this butter chicken curry, a dish that symbolises Indian food for millions of people all over the world

Ingredients

• 800g boneless and skinless chicken thighs, cut into bite-sized pieces

• coriander leaves, finely sliced red onion, sliced green or red chilli, naan bread or basmati rice, and chutney, to serve

For the marinade

• 120g Greek yogurt

• thumb-sized piece ginger, grated

• 4-5 garlic cloves, crushed

• 1 tbsp vegetable or coconut oil

• 1 lemon, juiced

• 3 tsp mild chilli powder

• 1 tsp ground cumin

- ½ tsp garam masala

- ½ tsp turmeric

For the sauce

- 1kg ripe vine or plum tomatoes

- thumb-sized piece ginger, peeled, half grated and half finely chopped

- 4 garlic cloves, crushed

- 4 green cardamom pods

- 2 cloves

- 1 bay leaf

- 1-2 tsp chilli powder

- 80g butter, diced

- 2 green chillies, cut lengthways

- 75ml single cream, plus a drizzle to serve

- 5-6 dried fenugreek leaves, crushed between your fingers (optional)

- 1 tsp garam masala

- 1 tbsp sugar or xylitol

For the spiced butter (optional)

- 3 tbsp ghee (see below) or butter

- 2 tsp black mustard seeds

- 1 dried whole Kashmiri chilli

- 6-8 dried curry leaves

Method

- STEP 1

Mix all of the marinade ingredients together in a large mixing bowl with 1½ tsp salt. Add the chicken pieces and mix together until well-coated, then cover the bowl and chill for 1 hr or overnight in the fridge.

- STEP 2

Heat the oven to 240C/220C fan/gas 9. Transfer the chicken pieces to a large baking tray (discard any remaining marinade), and cook for 10-15 mins. Turn the pieces after 10 mins so they colour evenly on both sides. The chicken doesn't need to be completely cooked through at this point as it will cook for a few more mins in the sauce.

• STEP 3

Meanwhile, for the sauce, slice the tomatoes in half and put in a large pan in a single layer with 125ml water, the grated ginger, garlic, cardamom, cloves and bay leaf. Simmer, covered, until the tomatoes have completely disintegrated, about 20-25 mins. Remove the whole spices and blend the tomato mixture with a stick blender, then pass it through a sieve to make a smooth purée. Return to a clean pan, add the chilli powder and simmer for 12-15 mins. It should slowly begin to thicken. When the sauce turns glossy, add the chicken pieces and any of the reserved roasting juices from the tray.

• STEP 4

Slowly stir in the butter, a couple of pieces at a time, and simmer for 6-8 mins until the chicken is cooked through. Add the chopped ginger, green chillies and cream, then simmer for a min or two longer, taking care that the sauce doesn't split. Stir in 1 tsp salt, fenugreek leaves, if using, and the garam masala, then check the seasoning, adjust if necessary, then add the sugar. In a separate pan, warm all the ingredients for the spiced butter, if using, until the seeds start to pop (see below). Spoon over the curry, scatter with the coriander, onion, chilli, and a drizzle more cream, if using. Serve with naan, pilau rice and chutney or keto bread for a keto-friendly version.

SMOKED HADDOCK WITH LEMON & DILL LENTILS

A low-GI supper for two with delicate fish and flavoured pulses - filling and nutritious

Ingredients

- 100g/ 4oz Puy lentils

- 1 small onion , finely chopped

- 1 carrot , finely chopped

- 1 celery stick, finely chopped

- 300ml/ ½ pint vegetable stock

- 1 rounded tbsp half-fat crème fraîche

- 2 tbsp chopped dill

- zest ½ lemon

- 2 x 100g/4oz smoked haddock fillets

- 50g/ 2oz baby spinach leaves

Method

- STEP 1

Tip the lentils into a pan with the onion, carrot and celery. Pour in the stock and bring to the boil. Give it a stir, then reduce the heat, cover and simmer for 20-25 mins, until the lentils are tender.

• STEP 2

Mix together the crème fraîche, half the dill and the lemon zest, adding a little seasoning. Put the fish in a shallow dish with a splash of water and cover with cling film. Microwave on Medium for 4-6 mins until the fish flakes easily.

• STEP 3

When the lentils are cooked, stir in the spinach until the leaves are barely wilted, then stir in the crème fraîche mixture. Divide between 2 warmed plates and top with the haddock. Scatter over the remaining dill and serve.

SPINACH, SWEET POTATO & LENTIL DHAL

A comforting vegan one-pot recipe that counts for 3 of your 5-a-day! You can't go wrong with this iron-rich, low-fat, low-calorie supper.

Ingredients

• 1 tbsp sesame oil

• 1 red onion, finely chopped

• 1 garlic clove, crushed

• thumb-sized piece ginger, peeled and finely chopped

• 1 red chilli, finely chopped

• 1½ tsp ground turmeric

• 1½ tsp ground cumin

• 2 sweet potatoes (about 400g/14oz), cut into even chunks

• 250g red split lentils

• 600ml vegetable stock

• 80g bag of spinach

- 4 spring onions, sliced on the diagonal, to serve

- ½ small pack of Thai basil, leaves torn, to serve

Method

- STEP 1

Heat 1 tbsp sesame oil in a wide-based pan with a tight-fitting lid.

- STEP 2

Add 1 finely chopped red onion and cook over a low heat for 10 mins, stirring occasionally, until softened.

- STEP 3

Add 1 crushed garlic clove, a finely chopped thumb-sized piece of ginger and 1 finely chopped red chilli, cook for 1 min, then add 1½ tsp ground turmeric and 1½ tsp ground cumin and cook for 1 min more.

- STEP 4

Turn up the heat to medium, add 2 sweet potatoes, cut into even chunks, and stir everything together so the potato is coated in the spice mixture.

• STEP 5

Tip in 250g red split lentils, 600ml vegetable stock and some seasoning.

• STEP 6

Bring the liquid to the boil, then reduce the heat, cover and cook for 20 mins until the lentils are tender and the potato is just holding its shape.

• STEP 7

Taste and adjust the seasoning, then gently stir in the 80g spinach. Once wilted, top with the 4 diagonally sliced spring onions and ½ small pack torn basil leaves to serve.

• STEP 8

Alternatively, allow to cool completely, then divide between airtight containers and store in the fridge for a healthy lunchbox.

OLD DELHI-STYLE BUTTER CHICKEN

Head to your spice rack to make this butter chicken curry, a dish that symbolises Indian food for millions of people all over the world

Ingredients

• 800g boneless and skinless chicken thighs, cut into bite-sized pieces

• coriander leaves, finely sliced red onion, sliced green or red chilli, naan bread or basmati rice, and chutney, to serve

For the marinade

• 120g Greek yogurt

• thumb-sized piece ginger, grated

• 4-5 garlic cloves, crushed

• 1 tbsp vegetable or coconut oil

• 1 lemon, juiced

• 3 tsp mild chilli powder

• 1 tsp ground cumin

- ½ tsp garam masala

- ½ tsp turmeric

For the sauce

- 1kg ripe vine or plum tomatoes

- thumb-sized piece ginger, peeled, half grated and half finely chopped

- 4 garlic cloves, crushed

- 4 green cardamom pods

- 2 cloves

- 1 bay leaf

- 1-2 tsp chilli powder

- 80g butter, diced

- 2 green chillies, cut lengthways

- 75ml single cream, plus a drizzle to serve

- 5-6 dried fenugreek leaves, crushed between your fingers (optional)

- 1 tsp garam masala

- 1 tbsp sugar or xylitol

For the spiced butter (optional)

- 3 tbsp ghee (see below) or butter

- 2 tsp black mustard seeds

- 1 dried whole Kashmiri chilli

- 6-8 dried curry leaves

Method

- STEP 1

Mix all of the marinade ingredients together in a large mixing bowl with 1½ tsp salt. Add the chicken pieces and mix together until well-coated, then cover the bowl and chill for 1 hr or overnight in the fridge.

- STEP 2

Heat the oven to 240C/220C fan/gas 9. Transfer the chicken pieces to a large baking tray (discard any remaining marinade), and cook for 10-15 mins. Turn the pieces after 10 mins so they colour evenly on both sides. The chicken doesn't need to be completely cooked through at this point as it will cook for a few more mins in the sauce.

• STEP 3

Meanwhile, for the sauce, slice the tomatoes in half and put in a large pan in a single layer with 125ml water, the grated ginger, garlic, cardamom, cloves and bay leaf. Simmer, covered, until the tomatoes have completely disintegrated, about 20-25 mins. Remove the whole spices and blend the tomato mixture with a stick blender, then pass it through a sieve to make a smooth purée. Return to a clean pan, add the chilli powder and simmer for 12-15 mins. It should slowly begin to thicken. When the sauce turns glossy, add the chicken pieces and any of the reserved roasting juices from the tray.

• STEP 4

Slowly stir in the butter, a couple of pieces at a time, and simmer for 6-8 mins until the chicken is cooked through. Add the chopped ginger, green chillies and cream, then simmer for a min or two longer, taking care that the sauce doesn't split. Stir in 1 tsp salt, fenugreek leaves, if using, and the garam masala, then check the seasoning, adjust if necessary, then add the sugar. In a separate pan, warm all the ingredients for the spiced butter, if using, until the seeds start to pop (see below). Spoon over the curry, scatter with the coriander, onion, chilli, and a drizzle more cream, if using. Serve with naan, pilau rice and chutney or keto bread for a keto-friendly version.

SALMON & LEEK PARCEL

A simple salmon dish, parcelled up to seal in the flavours. With creamy mascarpone and fresh leeks, this keto-friendly fish supper is easy and rich in omega-3

Ingredients

• 250g leek (about 3 small ones), thinly sliced

• 85g mascarpone

• 1 tbsp chopped dill , plus 1 tsp

• 2 skinless salmon fillets

• ½ lemon , grated zest of 1/4, plus a good squeeze of juice

• 2-3 tsp capers

• spinach wilted, to serve (optional)

Method

• STEP 1

Heat oven to 200C/180C fan/gas 6. Place two sheets of baking parchment (large enough to wrap up each salmon fillet) on your work surface.

• STEP 2

Put the leeks in a pan with 6 tbsp water, cover and bring to the boil. Cook for 5 mins until the water has been absorbed and the leeks are almost tender. Stir in the mascarpone, 1 tbsp dill and some seasoning.

• STEP 3

Spoon half the creamy leeks into the middle of one sheet of parchment and place a salmon fillet on top, then repeat to make a second parcel. Sprinkle over the lemon zest with a squeeze of juice, then scatter over the capers and the remaining 1 tsp dill.

• STEP 4

Bring the parchment up over the fish and join the two edges together by folding them over several times down the middle. Do the same with the ends and place the parcels, spaced apart, on a baking sheet.

• STEP 5

Bake for 12-15 mins, depending on how well done you like your fish, then carefully tear open the parcel. Serve with

lemon wedges for squeezing over and wilted spinach, if
you like.

SEEDED SODA BREAD WITH HUMMUS & TOMATOES

Pair our seeded soda bread with homemade hummus and tomatoes to start the day off with a low-GI option that will sustain you through the morning

Ingredients

- 1 tsp olive oil

- 8 x 80g portions cherry tomatoes, on or off the vine

- 12 slices seeded soda bread (see 'goes well with', below)

- 4 tsp four-seed mix (sunflower, pumpkin, sesame and golden flax seeds)

For the hummus

- 2 x 400g cans chickpeas

- 2 tbsp lemon juice

- 2-3 tsp ground coriander

- 1-2 tsp cumin

- 1 rounded tbsp tahini

• 2 tbsp extra virgin olive oil

Method

• STEP 1

First, make the hummus. Put all the ingredients in a bowl and blitz with a hand blender and 4 tbsp water from the canned chickpeas until smooth. Chill until needed.

• STEP 2

Heat the oil in a large non-stick frying pan, then add the whole cherry tomatoes in batches (on or off the vine) and cook over a medium heat for just a few minutes until they look on the point of bursting.

• STEP 3

To serve two for breakfast on the Healthy Diet Plan, toast 3 slices of the bread. Use a quarter of the hummus to spread over the toast, then top with a quarter of the tomatoes and scatter with ½ tsp of the seeds. Halve each slice of toast and serve 3 pieces per person. Keep the remaining bread, hummus and tomatoes chilled to serve on three subsequent mornings. Will keep chilled for up to four days.

LOW-FAT TURKEY BOLOGNESE

Swap your usual beef mince with turkey to reduce the fat content of this classic Italian sauce and serve with wholemeal pasta

Ingredients

• 400g lean turkey mince (choose breast instead of thigh mince if you can, as it has less fat)

• 2 tsp vegetable oil

• 1 large onion, chopped

• 1 large carrot, chopped

• 3 celery sticks, chopped

• 250g pack brown mushroom, finely chopped

• pinch of sugar

• 1 tbsp tomato purée

• 2 x 400g cans chopped tomato with garlic & herbs

• 400ml chicken stock, made from 1 low-sodium stock cube

• cooked wholemeal pasta and fresh basil leaves (optional), to serve

Method

• STEP 1

Heat a large non-stick frying pan and dry-fry the turkey mince until browned. Tip onto a plate and set aside.

• STEP 2

Add the oil and gently cook the onion, carrot and celery until softened, about 10 mins (add a splash of water if it starts to stick). Add the mushrooms and cook for a few mins, then add the sugar and tomato purée, and cook for 1 min more, stirring to stop it from sticking.

• STEP 3

Add the tomatoes, turkey and stock with some seasoning. Simmer for at least 20 mins (or longer) until thickened. Serve with the pasta and fresh basil, if you have it.

HEALTHY PEPPER, TOMATO & HAM OMELETTE

If you're in need of a healthy protein boost, try making this healthy omelette for breakfast – using fewer yolks lowers the cholesterol

Ingredients

• 2 whole eggs and 3 egg whites

• 1 tsp olive oil

• 1 red pepper, deseeded and finely chopped

• 2 spring onions, white and green parts kept separate, and finely chopped

• few slices wafer-thin extra-lean ham, shredded

• 25g reduced-fat mature cheddar

• wholemeal toast, to serve (optional)

• 1-2 chopped fresh tomatoes, to serve (optional)

Method

• STEP 1

Mix the eggs and egg whites with some seasoning and set aside. Heat the oil in a medium non-stick frying pan and cook the pepper for 3-4 mins. Throw in the white parts of the spring onions and cook for 1 min more. Pour in the eggs and cook over a medium heat until almost completely set.

• STEP 2

Sprinkle on the ham and cheese, and continue cooking until just set in the centre, or flash it under a hot grill if you like it more well done. Serve straight from the pan with the green part of the spring onions sprinkled on top, the chopped tomato and some wholemeal toast, if you like.

KERALAN CHICKEN COCONUT ISHTU

Anjum Anand adds green beans and spinach to this creamy chicken curry to make a flavourful one-pot meal - serve alongside rice, paratha, naan or rice noodles for a special supper. You can also make this keto-friendly by serving with cauliflower rice.

Ingredients

• 5 tbsp coconut oil or vegetable oil

• 5cm/2in cinnamon stick

• 6 green cardamom pods

• 4 cloves

• 10 black peppercorns , lightly crushed

• 1 star anise

• 15 curry leaves

• 1 medium onion , finely sliced

• thumb-sized piece of ginger , peeled and finely chopped

• 6 garlic cloves , finely chopped

• 2-3 green chillies

• 2 tsp fennel seeds

• ½ tsp ground turmeric

• 1 tbsp ground coriander

• 600g chicken thighs , skinned

• handful green beans , ends trimmed, halved if very long

• 400ml can coconut milk

• 2 tbsp coconut cream

• 1 tsp vinegar (or to taste)

• large handful baby spinach , blanched and water squeezed out

• small handful fresh coriander , to garnish

Method

• STEP 1

Heat the oil in a wide pan (a karahi or wok is ideal), then add the cinnamon stick, cardamom pods, cloves, peppercorns and star anise. Once the seeds have stopped popping, add the curry leaves and the onion and cook over a medium heat until translucent. Add the ginger, garlic and green chillies, and sauté gently for 1-2 mins or until the garlic is cooked.

• STEP 2

Grind the fennel seeds to a fine powder in a spice grinder or with a pestle and mortar, then add to the pan with the turmeric, ground coriander and a pinch of salt. Add a splash of water and cook for 2 mins. Put the chicken in the pan and cook in the spice paste for 2 mins. Add water to come a third of the way up the chicken, bring to a boil, then reduce the heat and cook, covered, for 1 hr, stirring occasionally.

• STEP 3

Once the liquid has reduced, add the green beans and coconut milk (including the thin milk that collects at the bottom of the can), cover and cook for another 10 mins. Uncover and cook off most of the excess liquid, stirring occasionally. Check the chicken is cooked all the way through. Stir in the coconut cream, vinegar and spinach, and bring to a simmer. Taste and adjust the seasoning, and serve topped with the coriander.

Fill up at breakfast time with this healthy low-sugar granola, served with your choice of milk and sliced fresh strawberries. It'll keep you going until lunch

Ingredients

• 200g rolled oats

• 150g bag mixed nuts

• 150g mixed seeds

• 1 orange , zested

• 2 tsp mixed spice

• 2 tsp cinnamon

• 2 tbsp cold pressed rapeseed oil

• 1½ tbsp maple syrup

Method

• STEP 1

Heat oven to 160C/140C fan/gas 4. Mix all the ingredients in a bowl with a pinch of salt, then spread out on a baking tray.

• STEP 2

Roast for 30-35 mins until golden, pulling the tray out of the oven twice while cooking to give everything a good stir – this will help the granola toast evenly. Leave to cool. Will keep in an airtight container for one month.

CAULIFLOWER RICE

Pulse cauliflower in a food processor to make cauliflower couscous or an easy rice-like side dish that's much lower GI and ready in just 10 minutes

Ingredients

- 1 medium cauliflower

- good handful coriander, chopped

- cumin seeds, toasted (optional)

Method

- STEP 1

Cut the hard core and stalks from the cauliflower and pulse the rest in a food processor to make grains the size of rice. Tip into a heatproof bowl, cover with cling film, then pierce and microwave for 7 mins on high – there is no need to add any water. Stir in the coriander. For spicier rice, add some toasted cumin seeds.

BURNT AUBERGINE VEGGIE CHILLI

This warming aubergine chilli is low fat and four of your five-a-day. Serve up this smoky spiced supper with brown rice and all your favourite trimmings

Ingredients

- 1 aubergine

- 1 tbsp olive oil or rapeseed oil

- 1 red onion, diced

- 2 carrots, finely diced

- 70g puy lentils or green lentils, rinsed

- 30g red lentils, rinsed

- 400g can kidney beans

- 3 tbsp dark soy sauce

- 400g can chopped tomatoes

- 20g dark chocolate, finely chopped

- ¼ tsp chilli powder

- 2 tsp dried oregano

- 2 tsp ground cumin

- 2 tsp sweet smoked paprika

- 1 tsp coriander

- 1 tsp cinnamon

- 800ml vegetable stock

- ½ lime, juiced

To serve

- brown rice

- tortilla chips, mashed avocado, yogurt or soured cream, grated cheddar, roughly chopped coriander (optional)

Method

- STEP 1

If you have a gas hob, put the aubergine directly onto a lit ring to char completely, turning occasionally with kitchen tongs, until burnt all over. Alternatively, use a barbecue or heat the grill to its highest setting and cook, turning occasionally, until completely blackened (the grill won't give you the same smoky flavour). Set aside to cool on a plate, then peel off the charred skin and remove the stem. Roughly chop the flesh and set aside.

• STEP 2

In a large pan, heat the oil, add the onion and carrots with a pinch of salt, and fry over a low-medium heat for 15-20 mins until the carrots have softened.

• STEP 3

Add the aubergine, both types of lentils, the kidney beans with the liquid from the can, soy sauce, tomatoes, chocolate, chilli powder, oregano and the spices. Stir to combine, then pour in the stock. Bring to the boil, then turn down the heat to very low. Cover with a lid and cook for 1½ hrs, checking and stirring every 15-20 mins to prevent it from burning.

• STEP 4

Remove the lid and let the mixture simmer over a low-medium heat, stirring occasionally, for about 15 mins until you get a thick sauce. Stir in the lime juice and taste for seasoning – add more salt if needed. Serve hot over rice with whichever accompaniments you want!

BUTTERNUT SQUASH & CHICKPEA TAGINE

Make this tasty vegetarian tagine that kids will love as much as grown-ups. It's a great way to serve four of their five-a-day and it's freezeable

Ingredients

• 1tbsp oil

• 1 red onion, finely chopped

• 2 garlic cloves, crushed

• 1tsp grated ginger

• ground cumin

• 1tsp ground coriander

• 1tsp cinnamon

• mild chilli powder

• 450g bag frozen butternut squash chunks

• 2 carrots, cut into small dice

• 1 courgette, cut into small dice

• chopped tomatoes

• chickpeas, drained

• cooked couscous or rice, to serve

Method

• STEP 1

Heat the oil in a heavy-based pan, then slowly cook the onions for around 10 mins until starting to caramelise. Stir in the garlic, ginger and spices and cook for a further 2 mins. Add the vegetables and canned tomatoes and bring to a simmer. Put the lid on and simmer for around 15 mins or until all the veg are tender. Stir in the chickpeas, heat through and serve with couscous or rice.

LOW-FAT CHICKEN BIRYANI

This fragrant Indian chicken curry with rice topping has half the fat of your normal takeaway, and it's low calorie

Ingredients

• 3 garlic cloves , finely grated

• 2 tsp finely grated ginger

• ¼ tsp ground cinnamon

• 1 tsp turmeric

• 5 tbsp natural yogurt

• 600g boneless, skinless chicken breast , cut into 4-5cm pieces

• 2 tbsp semi-skimmed milk

• good pinch saffron

• 4 medium onions

• 4 tbsp rapeseed oil

• ½ tsp hot chilli powder

• 1 cinnamon stick , broken in half

• 5 green cardamom pods , lightly bashed to split

• 3 cloves

• 1 tsp cumin seed

• 280g basmati rice

• 700ml chicken stock

• 1 tsp garam masala

• handful chopped coriander leaves

Method

• STEP 1

In a mixing bowl, stir together the garlic, ginger, cinnamon, turmeric and yogurt with some pepper and ¼ tsp salt. Tip in the chicken pieces and stir to coat (see step 1, above). Cover and marinate in the fridge for about 1 hr or longer if you have time. Warm the milk to tepid, stir in the saffron and set aside.

• STEP 2

Heat oven to 200C/180C fan/gas 6. Slice each onion in half lengthways, reserve half and cut the other half into thin slices. Pour 1½ tbsp of the oil onto a baking tray, scatter over the sliced onion, toss to coat, then spread out in a thin, even layer (step 2). Roast for 40-45 mins, stirring halfway, until golden.

• STEP 3

When the chicken has marinated, thinly slice the reserved onion. Heat 1 tbsp oil in a large sauté or frying pan. Fry the onion for 4-5 mins until golden. Stir in the chicken, a spoonful at a time, frying until it is no longer opaque, before adding the next spoonful (this helps to prevent the yogurt from curdling). Once the last of the chicken has been added, stir-fry for a further 5 mins until everything looks juicy. Scrape any sticky bits off the bottom of the pan, stir in the chilli powder, then pour in 100ml water, cover and simmer on a low heat for 15 mins. Remove and set aside.

• STEP 4

Cook the rice while the chicken simmers. Heat another 1 tbsp oil in a large sauté pan, then drop in the cinnamon stick, cardamom, cloves and cumin seeds. Fry briefly until their aroma is released. Tip in the rice (step 3) and fry for

1 min, stirring constantly. Stir in the stock and bring to the boil. Lower the heat and simmer, covered, for about 8 mins or until all the stock has been absorbed. Remove from the heat and leave with the lid on for a few mins, so the rice can fluff up. Stir the garam masala into the remaining 1½ tsp oil and set aside. When the onions are roasted, remove and reduce oven to 180C/160C fan/gas 4.

• STEP 5

Spoon half the chicken and its juices into an ovenproof dish, about 25 x 18 x 6cm, then scatter over a third of the roasted onions. Remove the whole spices from the rice, then layer half of the rice over the chicken and onions. Drizzle over the spiced oil. Spoon over the rest of the chicken and a third more onions. Top with the remaining rice (step 4) and drizzle over the saffron-infused milk. Scatter over the rest of the onions, cover tightly with foil and heat through in the oven for about 25 mins. Serve scattered with the mint and coriander.

RED LENTIL, CHICKPEA & CHILLI SOUP

Come home to a warming bowlful of this filling, low-fat soup

Ingredients

• 2 tsp cumin seeds

• large pinch chilli flakes

• 1 tbsp olive oil

• 1 red onion, chopped

• 140g red split lentils

• 850ml vegetable stock or water

• 400g can tomatoes, whole or chopped

• 200g can chickpeas or ½ a can, drained and rinsed (freeze leftovers)

• small bunch coriander, roughly chopped (save a few leaves, to serve)

• 4 tbsp 0% Greek yogurt, to serve

Method

• STEP 1

Heat a large saucepan and dry-fry 2 tsp cumin seeds and a large pinch of chilli flakes for 1 min, or until they start to jump around the pan and release their aromas.

• STEP 2

Add 1 tbsp olive oil and 1 chopped red onion, and cook for 5 mins.

• STEP 3

Stir in 140g red split lentils, 850ml vegetable stock or water and a 400g can tomatoes, then bring to the boil. Simmer for 15 mins until the lentils have softened.

• STEP 4

Whizz the soup with a stick blender or in a food processor until it is a rough purée, pour back into the pan and add a 200g can drained and rinsed chickpeas.

• STEP 5

Heat gently, season well and stir in a small bunch of chopped coriander, reserving a few leaves to serve. Finish with 4 tbsp 0% Greek yogurt and extra coriander leaves.

Barley has a low Gi, so it will leave you feeling fuller for longer. You'll get two of your five-a-day from this hearty salad, too

Ingredients

• 2 tbsp olive oil

• 2 garlic cloves , finely chopped

• pinch dried chilli flakes

• small bunch mint , chopped

• 2 lean lamb leg steaks, about 100g/4oz each, trimmed of any fat

• 100g pearl barley

• 200g broad beans , fresh or frozen, podded and skins removed, if you like

• 100g frozen petits pois

• 1 small red onion , finely chopped

• zest and juice 1 lemon

Method

• STEP 1

Mix together 1 tbsp oil, the garlic, chilli, half the mint and some salt and pepper. Rub all over the steaks, then if you have time, leave to marinate for up to 2 hrs.

• STEP 2

Cook the pearl barley in boiling, salted water until tender, but not too soft, about 20 mins. Cook the beans and peas in the same pan for the last 2 mins. Drain really well, then tip into a large bowl. Add the red onion, remaining mint, lemon zest and juice, remaining oil, salt and pepper. Toss everything together.

• STEP 3

Heat a griddle or frying pan until almost smoking and cook the lamb for 4 mins on each side for pink, or longer if you prefer your meat well done. Divide the barley salad between 2 plates and serve with the grilled lamb, drizzled with any pan juices

CONCLUSION

In order for you to maintain your current weight, you need to burn as many calories as you consume. To lose weight, you need to burn more calories than you consume. Weight loss is best done with a combination of reducing calories in your diet and increasing your physical activity and exercise. Selecting foods based on a glycemic index or glycemic load value may help you manage your weight because many foods that should be included in a well-balanced, low-fat, healthy diet with minimally processed foods — whole-grain products, fruits, vegetables and low-fat dairy products — have low-GI values.

For some people, a commercial low-GI diet may provide needed direction to help them make better choices for a healthy diet plan. The researchers who maintain the GI database caution, however, that the "glycemic index should not be used in isolation" and that other nutritional factors — calories, fat, fiber, vitamins and other nutrients — should be considered.